Juicing For
A Juicing Book With the Best Juicing Recipes to Help You Lose Weight and Gain Energy

Praise For Juicing For Weight Loss:

"I was looking for a juicing book with the basics of juicing, along with recipes and their health benefits, and I found it all in this awesome book! I wanted to find a way to get more nutrition into my body than I could by just eating raw fruits and veggies, and I wanted to lose weight, in a healthy way. This book helped me do all that! I love the recipes - Detox Cleanser, Energy Blaster, Fat Buster ... delicious recipes that help you gain the most from your fruits and vegetables. I would recommend this book to all!"
- Monica E. ★★★★★

"I would recommend this book to those wanting to learn about juicing. I like how it is condensed and not over the top crazy like some of the other books out there. I've been sticking to the recipes outlined in the book and I am feeling a ton better."

- Robert K. ★★★★★

"I really think this book does a good job explaining what it takes to get the most out of juicing. Especially for those looking to start the new year healthier (like me)."
- Brittany R. ★★★★★

"This book really did a good job explaining why juicing isn't a diet. It's more of a lifestyle and I'm sticking to it everyday!"
- Susan B. ★★★★★

About The Author:

Ryan E. Taylor is a former professional athlete and a serious health advocate. He writes his books in order to inspire others to live a healthier lifestyle full of energy and vitality. His hope is that you take something from this book, apply it to your life, and begin to transform your body, mind, and spirit.

More Amazon Best Sellers That Compliment Juicing:

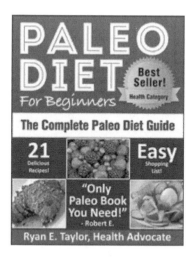

Go Here -- FCRW.org/paleo

Copyright © 2012-2013 - All rights reserved.

Paperback/Hardcover ISBN 978-0-9893135-6-8

Table of Contents

Introduction

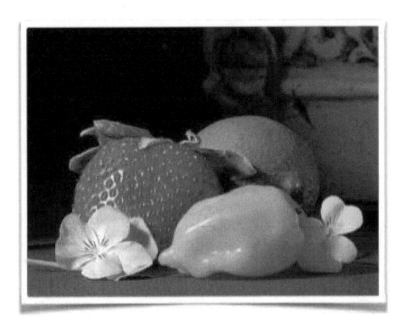

Congratulations and thank you for your decision to purchase this juicing e-book! You may not know it yet, but you've just taken the most important step to getting your health and vitality back! As I always say... juicing is life! Literally, the minerals and vitamins you consume from whole, raw, natural fruits and vegetables produce life - and life more abundantly! We are all organic living beings and it's important to put organic living foods into our bodies.

I am sure you're going to thoroughly enjoy the multitude of benefits that will come from consuming more fresh fruits and vegetables in your daily diet through juicing.

Included in this book is a variety of different juicing recipes.   But I want to make one thing clear - juicing is not an exact science, and your creativity can also play a big part in it. There are no definitive set rules to what you can and cannot mix when juicing vegetables and fruits (aside from a few non- "juice-able" produce items).

So, essentially, the sky is the limit! I have made this juicing e-book as straightforward as possible because I don't want to overwhelm you with a ton of technical mumbo jumbo - just the facts you need to start losing weight with a juicing lifestyle. I firmly believe in two lifestyle choices that will have the most impact on your health and overall well-being... Juicing and The Paleo Diet. This book will strictly focus on juicing, however, I strongly encourage you to take a look at The Paleo Diet as well (if you haven't already!)

Food For Thought:

Throughout this book I may mention the word "diet." When I use the word "diet" I'm not referring to juicing in the same category as one

of those gimmicky diets... you know - Atkins, South Beach, Low Carb, etc. I say diet in the literal sense of the word, as in your daily eating routine.

I want you to remember this concept because at the end of the day, I want juicing to be fun! Use this book as a guide, but in all honesty... go nuts! :-) We've included a chart in this book that will allow you to see which fruits and vegetables are the best for juicing. Within those guidelines you can mix-and-match all day long.

My Juicing Story

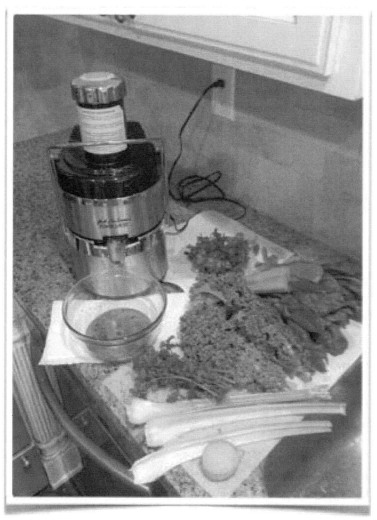

I've always been somewhat healthy (or so I thought), but it wasn't until I started juicing that I realized the full potential my body had in store for me. I didn't think I was a horrible eater... I would have the occasional pasta, one piece of bread at dinner, and diet soda (which had to be healthier, right?). BUT... I never felt 100% healthy, energetic, and full of life - that is, until I found the power of juicing and the amazing way it made me feel each and every day I did it.

Juicing always seemed like something weird hippie people did (no offense to hippies). I couldn't see the full benefit of taking a fruit or vegetable, sticking it into a machine, and drinking the juice. I thought it was a waste of time and I didn't think it could actually do anything for my body. But boy, was I wrong!

I quickly learned that juicing is a more efficient way of getting the nutrients and antioxidant properties into your system without the hassle of digestion. Think about it, when you eat a fruit or vegetable, it takes a lot of energy to chew, swallow, allow your stomach to process, and then finally dispose of the parts you don't need. In essence, juicing provides a faster way to rapidly absorb all the health benefits you need from fresh fruit and vegetables, without the hassle of the digestion process! Makes sense, right? Vitamins, antioxidants, and other health properties are allowed to immediately enter your blood stream, allowing for much faster results!

So...What is Juicing?

At its simplest form, juicing is the practice of extracting the juice from vegetables and/or fruits and discarding the solid portion of the vegetable or fruit. The process involves using an electronic or manual machine to extract the juice from vegetables or fruits, and has been used for quite some time now. That being said, it has only recently taken off as a legitimate way to revitalize the body, gain more energy, lose weight, detox, and so much more.

Juicing is an excellent way to obtain a variety of vitamins, including: vitamin A, vitamin C, vitamin B Complex and vitamin E, just to name a few. Any benefits that a person can obtain from eating vegetables can be obtained from the juicing process, but like I mentioned earlier, you should still consume whole fruits and vegetables to maintain fiber throughout your diet.

There are also recommendations for juice combinations that will address certain conditions. For instance, juices may help people with anemia, weight loss, osteoporosis, cataracts, insomnia, allergies, hair loss and dandruff. If you follow the recipes, juicing can truly be beneficial and helpful to your health.

Food For Thought:

**Important Information About Sweeteners:
We in no way recommend using artificial
sweeteners!**

**Some recipes in this book may recommend
Agave as a sweetener. We have included a
sweetener conversion chart for you that
includes stevia, agave, sugar, and honey. We use
these sweeteners as our top picks ONLY if you
really need them. Otherwise, I recommend
going all-natural as much as possible. It is also
good to note that fruit can be used as a good all-
natural sweetener.**

Sugar Table
1 c. Sugar = 1 tsp Stevia or Liquid
1 c. Sugar = 2/3 c. Agave
1 c. Sugar = 1/2 c. Honey

Produce List

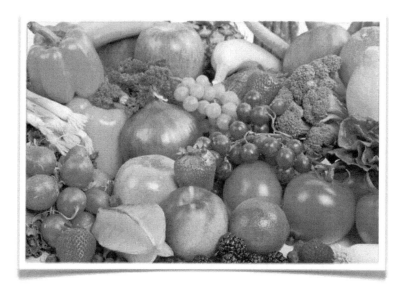

Use the following chart to help you decide how to mix-and-match the best produce for juicing.

Note: All of these produce items can be juiced. I am giving you a quick reference guide as to what items are ideal for juicing and which ones you may find a little more challenging. For example, kale is a little tougher to juice but I almost always include it in my juicing routine. Tip: When juicing a leafy vegetable such as kale, always follow it up with something that contains A LOT of juice (i.e., celery, cucumber, apple, etc.).

Fruits and Vegetables Ideal For Juicing

Apple
Asparagus
Brussels sprouts
Cabbage
Cantaloupe
Celery
Cherry (pitted)
Clementine
Cranberry
Cucumber
Fennel
Ginger
Grapefruit
Grape
Guava
Honeydew melon
Horse radish
Kiwi
Lemon
Lettuce
Lime
Nectarine
Onion
Orange
Peach
Pear (firm)
Peppers

Pineapple
Pomegranate
Pumpkin
Radish
Squash
Strawberry
Tangerine
Tomato
Watermelon

Fruits and Vegetables More Challenging To Juice (But Still Great For You)

Apricot
Basil
Beet
Blackberry
Blueberry
Broccoli
Carrot
Cauliflower
Collard Green
Dandelion Green
Endive
Green Bean
Green Pea
Kale
Leafy Greens
Mango

Mint
Mushroom
Okra
Papaya
Parsley
Passion Fruit
Peppermint
Plum
Raspberry
Spinach
Swiss Chard
Turnip
Watercress
Wheatgrass

Fruits and Vegetables Containing A Lot of Juice

Apple
Cantaloupe
Celery
Clementine
Cranberry
Cucumber
Grapefruit
Grape
Honeydew melon
Lemon
Lime
Orange

Peppers
Pineapple
Tangerine
Tomato
Watermelon

Juicing No-Nos

While the previous chart hopefully gives you a base for which produce items juice the best, there are certain fruits and veggies that are not a good match for juicing. Examples of these items are avocados, bananas, and coconut. However, we DO recommend eating these foods whole, as they are high in nutrition and can add to your diet in an extremely beneficial way.

Always try to rid your fruits of their pits or seeds, as these don't provide nutritional value and some may contain ingredients that may irritate your stomach. Also, never use the green tops of rhubarb (the oxalic acid in the leaves is toxic).

Do not add water or liquid to your juicer either... other than that, have at it!!

Juice and Pulp Yield Per Produce

Apples
6 medium apples = 2 c. juice
6 medium apples = 1 1/2 c. pulp

Pears
6 medium pears = 2 c. juice

6 medium pears = 1 1/2 c. pulp

Carrots
5 large carrots = 1 c. juice
5 large carrots = 1 1/2 c. pulp

Celery Stalks
4 celery stalks = 3/4 c. juice
4 celery stalks = 1/4 c. pulp

Cucumbers
1 large cucumber= 1 c. juice
1 large cucumber= 1/3 c. pulp

Mangoes
6 mangoes = 2 1/2 c. juice
6 mangoes = 2 c. pulp

Oranges
5 med. oranges= 2 c. juice
5 med. oranges= 1 1/2 c. pulp

Pineapples
2 med. pineapples = 2 c. juice
2 med. pineapples = 2 1/2 c. pulp

Potatoes
8 med. red potatoes = 2 1/2 c. juice
8 med. red potatoes = 2 c. pulp

Raspberries

1/2 pt. raspberries = 1/2 c. juice
1/2 pt. raspberries = 1/4 c. pulp

Strawberries
30 strawberries = 2 c. juice
30 strawberries = 1/3 c. pulp

Juicing Overview

Juicing has moved into the mainstream, and more people are noticing that they can increase their health by simply drinking fresh fruit and vegetable juice every day. From juice bars in local shopping centers to home juicing machines, it has never been easier to get the recommended daily amount of fruits and vegetables.

The average person living in the United States only eats about 1 ½ servings of vegetables a day, and little to no fruit. The National Cancer Institute recommends a daily intake of at least 5 vegetables and 3 fruits a day; therefore, making a fresh juice is an easy way to get all of the recommended daily amounts quickly and easily. In fact, one juice can provide most or all the recommended amount of vitamins for an entire day. Mixing the fruit with veggies makes for a sweet juice that even the kids will love.

Since juicing machines separate the fiber from the rest of the fruits and vegetables, all that is left is the delicious vitamins and nutrients. A person can drink a lot more fruits and veggies than they can eat when whole. This means the body is getting much more vitamins and nutrients into the body.

Citrus fruits have a high vitamin C content. Carrot juice contains a healthy portion of vitamin A, and green leafy vegetables like kale and spinach are an excellent source of vitamin E. Add a few fruits to a juice, like apples and oranges to get essential minerals, including potassium, iron, iodine, copper, and magnesium, and other vital vitamins. The blood can easily absorb all these nutrients because there is no fiber that must be digested first.

Disease Prevention

Drinking a green juice every morning, on an empty stomach so the body can absorb as much of the vitamins and minerals as possible, has shown to reduce the risk of cancer and other diseases. Scientists are now looking at fruits and vegetables to try and isolate the chemicals in these foods that seem to prevent illness, like the phytochemicals in broccoli that may cure breast cancer, or the phytochemicals in grapes that appear to protect the DNA in every individual cell of the body.

These are just a few of the wonderful benefits of juicing. The health benefits are the biggest reason anyone should add fresh fruit and vegetable juice to their diet every day. It is an inexpensive way to reduce the risk of disease and improve your quality of life.

Why is Juicing Important?

Juicing is important for busy people who have a difficult time consuming the recommended daily amounts of fruits and vegetables, or for anyone else who wants to take their health to the next level. A single juice or vegetable drink can account for the recommended daily amount of nutrients and vitamins the body needs to thrive. Nutrients help the body heal and fight free radicals.

Juicing can also help with colon cleansing and detoxification (which we'll go over shortly). It is important to remove harmful toxins from the body that may be trapped in the colon or liver. Detoxifying the body can help to fight cancer and help to cleanse the body of other toxins.

Minor Disadvantages of Juicing

There are three disadvantages to juicing, but the disadvantages do not outweigh the benefits:

Juicing raises insulin levels when the liquid is consumed. (This may be a problem for diabetics.) Juicing can be time-consuming if you are used to fast food.

Juicing typically needs to be consumed immediately after the juicing process to get the most benefit from the nutrients.

That being said, it is important to know that juicing is worth every ounce of effort and time it takes to make the juice. Everything is about routines and if you get in the routine of juicing. it simply becomes part of your day. This will allow you to form an ongoing ritual of consuming fresh fruits and vegetables each and every day.

Types of Juicers

The type of juicer you choose will make a slight difference in the healthiness of the juice extracted from the fruits and vegetables, but it is important to know that you don't need to go crazy over which juicer to use. The difference between most juicers is the amount of heat and friction they cause. Heat detracts from the health benefits of the juice so the less heat used the more nutrients are preserved. Certain juicers can, however, control the amount of heat produced. Here are three different types of juicers available:

Masticating Juicer - Masticating juicers produce a healthier juice than the centrifugal juicer. This type of juicer uses a masticating motion to grind and extract the juice. Masticating juicers can also make baby foods, fruit desserts and nut butters.

Centrifugal Juicer - (This is the first juicer I owned and it did the job just fine.) Most affordable juicers are centrifugal. This type of juicer puts fruits and vegetables in close contact with a high-speed spinning shredder. The pulp remains in the shredder, and the juice passes through the basket. This type of juicer can make juice for one to two people at a time, or one quart of juice.

Triturating Juicer - The healthiest juice is extracted using a triturating, or twin-gear, juicer. The twin-gear juicer operates at a lower speed. Because the machine generates less heat, the juice is able to retain more nutrients, thus leading some to believe that this type of juicer creates a healthier juice. These juicers are more expensive and start at approximately $400 to $800.

Recommendation: If money isn't an issue, go for the masticating juicer. It uses gears and keeps your juice in its optimal state. However, if you are on a budget, a centrifugal juicer will do just fine. My very first juicer was a basic Jack LaLanne that I got for under $100 and it works like a charm.

Juicing for Weight Loss and Energy - Phase 1 (Detoxing)

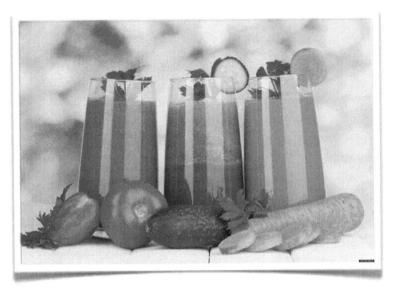

Before embarking on any new diet or cleanse, it is always recommended that a physician be consulted for any change lasting more than three days. Anyone with health challenges should consult a doctor prior to starting any juice cleanse. While eating fruits and vegetables is generally considered a positive health habit, any diet that does not include protein, or is radically different, can have negative health repercussions for certain people. The first step in juicing for weight loss is the most important, and we will spend the majority of the time going over what to expect in your detox phase (phase 1).

Juicing for weight loss isn't an exact science. There are essentially two easy phases, or steps - the detox phase and the maintenance/routine phase. We will start with the first phase... Detoxing. At the core, detoxing through juicing is the cleansing of the colon, gallbladder, kidneys, and digestive tract. It is important to start with a cleanse in order to flush your body and rid it of the toxins that create buildup and hostile environments within your cells.

Weight loss is able to occur when your body is flushed of these toxins, and a "clean slate" is started within your digestive tract. When your body cleanses its organs and cleanses the digestive tract, you're able to process foods a lot easier, making digestion a lot easier. When your digestive system is clean and working properly, buildup becomes less frequent, and allows you to get food in and out of your body while absorbing the majority of beneficial vitamins and nutrients. Your body then starts to kick into the proper gear and everything from there gets better. Your metabolism gets faster and you have more energy, thus allowing you to burn calories more efficiently!

The concept of juicing for weight loss really is quite simple. It works extremely well when coupled with a whole food diet devoid of "nasty" foods such as carbs and sugar. After the cleanse portion, you will then be able to incorporate juicing into your normal diet, and continue a healthy lifestyle that will allow you to lose weight (but more importantly, fat).

Preparing For A Cleanse

A juice cleanse is not something to mess around with. It can be very beneficial to your body, but you have to start off on the right track. Two days before you begin your cleanse, I recommend that you begin to eliminate processed foods (this includes fast food).

Before a cleanse starts, you should stick to fruits, vegetables, and lean proteins such as chicken and fish. You may even notice a difference eating this way for the first couple days before your cleanse starts. It is important that you do this because you want to "prime the pump" in order to get your body ready to get rid of the toxins within your cells.

I'd also recommend you eliminate soda, sugary drinks, and stimulants such as caffeine and coffee. This means no energy drinks or your daily latte at your favorite coffee joint. Don't worry! After the cleanse you can go back to doing what you want to do. But I have a sneaking suspicion that you may want to stay on track and eat a lot healthier! (Totally up to you, though.)

A juice cleanse is different from fasting because you are still giving your body all of the necessary vitamins and nutrients, while allowing your overall digestive system to take a break from the daily grind of solid foods.

The goal here is to drink your juices without the consumption of food, which allows you to take in the appropriate nutrients for the day but also with a limited number of calories. Detoxing is one of the most important things you can do for your body. With a juice-cleansing detox, you are essentially ridding the body of foreign chemicals and heavy metals. It's also important to know that even our own cells create toxins within the body.

Typically toxins can build up and affect us in many ways. Many of these elements and symptoms are as follows: (Do you experience any of these?)

Constipation
Tissue inflammation
Fatigue
Multiple allergies
Repeated illnesses
Minor or severe depression
Trouble sleeping or insomnia

IBS or irritable bowel syndrome

If you suffer from any of these symptoms, a juice cleanse might be the best way to go! A juice cleanse can gently help your body eliminate toxins and restore balance to your entire body. Our bodies need a little help to jump-start the flushing of our systems. When we consume fresh fruits and vegetables, the enzymes are able to go into overdrive, and help to replenish the supply that is usually taken from our organs in order to digest most of the food we put into our bodies each and every day.

What To Expect During A Cleanse

Detoxing is an essential part of having a healthy diet, and you should do it on a regular basis. However, it is also important to know that with any detox program, you are ridding your body of the harmful chemicals and damaged cells so there might be a chance of your body feeling different than it usually does. Your body isn't used to getting such an overdose of essential vitamins and minerals, and the "cleaning" process can vary in intensity depending on how often you detox and how good your diet is.

There is nothing to be afraid of! This simply means that you might experience a few symptoms that are less than enjoyable. But let me remind you... this is a great thing! It means your body is actually doing something good for itself and repairing and restoring you to the person you were created to be.

Some symptoms you may experience during a juice detox are:

Nausea
Fatigue
Increased moodiness
Sore muscles
Weakness
Diarrhea
Sore throat
Fever
Lack of appetite
Headaches

REMEMBER, these are just a few symptoms that are sometimes associated with a cleanse. The most common symptoms during a cleanse are intense thirst and mild stomach ache. This occurs because your body is flushing out your digestive tract and ridding it of unwanted toxins. This creates an environment that your body is not used to.

Note: I only include these symptoms just in case they occur. If they do occur it is important to see a physician right away. That being said, you should be fine and all should go according to plan.

The following recipes (and all recipes in this book) are meant to serve as a guide for your juicing adventure. Most of my recipes are perfect for cleansing the body of toxic cells, and most were designed to give you an energy boost.

Phase 1 Juicing Recipes

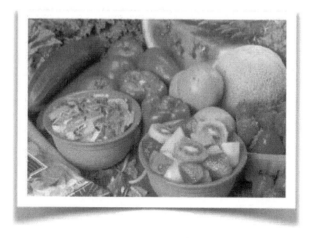

Please be aware that we add nutritional info for informational purposes, and these figures are just rough estimates. That being said, if you stick to the veggie and fruit chart in the beginning of the book, you don't need to worry about nutritional info at all. Juicing is extremely healthy for your body when done the right way. Enjoy!

Note: A lot of juicing books offer "tons" of recipes - this is done mainly for marketing purposes. I don't care about that stuff. What I care about is giving you tried and true recipes that have been tested by many others like you and me. I also encourage testing different recipes using mine as a guide. Maybe take an ingredient out or substitute one with another.

Energy Blaster

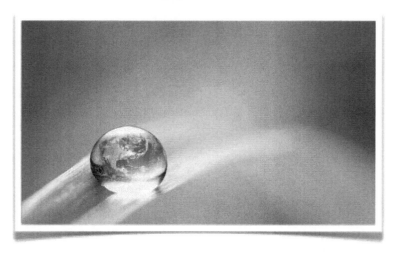

This juice will help energize you and get you out of bed on those days you just can't find the energy to get your day started. It'll refresh you and energize you - but more importantly, it'll detox you. :-)

Start to finish time: 10 minutes

Difficulty: Easy

Yield: (1) 8-oz. glass

Ingredients:
3 to 4 carrots, washed, ends removed
1 peeled cucumber

1/2 beetroot, leaves removed and washed
1/2 lemon peel
1-inch piece ginger root, scrubbed and peeled if
necessary

Instructions:
Cut carrots, cucumber, and beetroot in small
enough chunks to fit in the juicer's feed tube, then
process.
Put lemon and ginger root into juicer feed.
After juicing ingredients, pour into the glass and
add ice if desired.

Nutritional info:
Calories: 142
Total Fat: 2.7g
Total Carbohydrates: 17.9g
Dietary Fiber: 2.9g
Sugars: 8.5g
Protein: 0.9g
Sodium: 0.13 mg

Mean and Green Cleanse

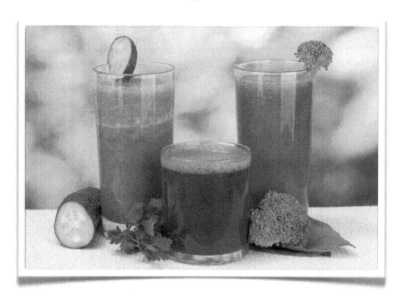

This juice cleanse will help rid the liver and gallbladder of toxins by flooding them with vitamins and nutrients that you might not be getting in your daily diet. It is important to note that you can mix-and-match ingredients as long as you keep the base ingredients the same.

Start to finish time: 5 minutes

Difficulty Level: Easy

Yield: (1) 8-oz. glass

Ingredients:
1 handful of parsley, washed
4 medium carrots, greens removed, washed, ends trimmed
1 small beetroot (leafy portion removed)
2 celery stalks with greens, washed and ends trimmed
1/2 lemon, peeled

Instructions:
Process washed parsley into juicer.
Feed carrots, beetroots with leaves, celery, and peeled lemon into juicer.
Pour juice into a glass. Add ice if desired.
Drink immediately.

Nutritional info:
Calories: 157
Total Fat: 3.2g
Total Carbohydrates: 21.8g
Dietary Fiber: 3.8g
Sugars: 11.8g
Protein: 2.3g
Sodium: 2mg

Full-Body Detox

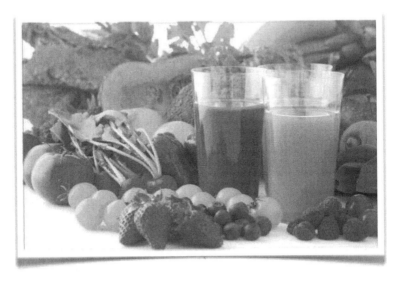

This is one of the best ways to do a full-body detox. Even if you are not in the process of detoxing, you should still use this recipe at least once every three days. Ideally (if possible), it would be great to do this juice every other day.

Start to finish time: 10 minutes

Difficulty Level: Easy

Yield: (1) 8-oz. glass

Ingredients:
1 tomato, washed

1 medium asparagus spear, washed
1 cucumber, washed and peeled
½ lemon, peeled, ice optional

Instructions:
Process tomato, asparagus, cucumber, and lemon into your juicer.
Pour into a glass, and serve with ice if desired.

Nutritional info:
Calories: 51.5
Total Fat: 0.78g
Total Carbohydrates: 11.2g
Dietary Fiber: 3.6g
Sugars: 6.2g
Protein: 2.6g
Sodium: 10mg

Liver Blaster

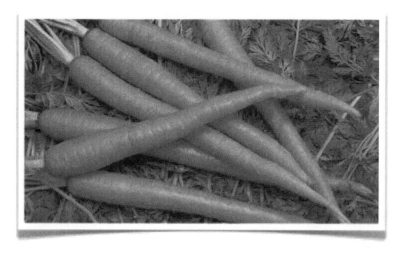

This juicing recipe is designed specifically to help cleanse and support your liver. The liver plays a vital role in the digestion process, as well as your metabolism. It is one of the most important organs in the human body so there is good reason to treat it right. The purpose of this juice is to help cleanse the liver and get it working in its optimal state.

Start to finish time: 10 minutes

Difficulty Level: Easy

Yield: (1) 8-oz. glass

Ingredients:

1 handful of dandelion (optional, but recommended)
3-4 carrots, washed and peeled
1/2 cucumber, peeled
1/2 lemon, peeled

Instructions:
Cut carrots and cucumbers into smaller pieces and feed into your juicer.
Add the dandelion to juicer (if using).
Add lemon to the juicer.
After juicing, pour into a glass. Add ice if desired.

Nutritional info:
Calories: 132
Total Fat: 1.2g
Total Carbohydrates: 30.5g
Dietary Fiber: 9.1g
Sugars: 15.1g
Protein: 3.2g
Sodium: 172mg

The Fave

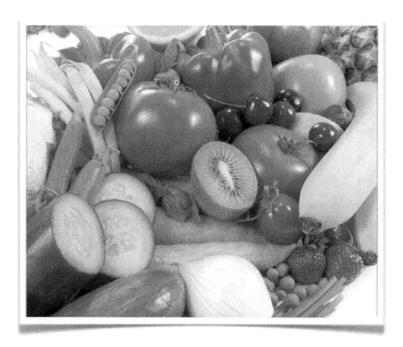

This is one of my favorite juicing recipes because it is easy, but it also packs a punch. It's full of healthy vitamins, and the ingredients are usually easy to find and in season. It's just what I like - simple and effective.

Start to finish time: 10 minutes

Difficulty Level: Easy

Yield: (1) 8-oz. glass

Ingredients:
2 large carrots
2 cups of kale
2 medium Granny Smith apples
1 medium tomato
¼-inch ginger

Instructions:
Feed kale into the juicer first, and then add carrots and Granny Smith apples.
Add ginger.
Add tomato.
After juicing, pour into a glass. Add ice if desired.

Nutritional info:
Calories: 102
Total Fat: 1.6g
Total Carbohydrates: 20.5g
Dietary Fiber: 9.1g
Sugars: 15.1g
Protein: 3.2g
Sodium: 122mg

The Smorgasbord

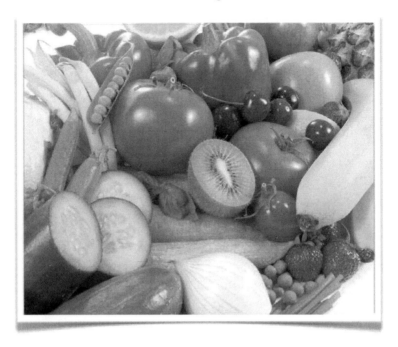

This cleanse is made up of a variety of different fruits and vegetables, all of which will flush your system and allow detoxification to take place. The only downfall of this cleanse is that it requires a variety of fruits and vegetables. It is important to note that with this cleanse, you may experience a slight stomach ache (goes away after a little bit), only because the juice is making its way through your GI tract and cleaning your system.

Ingredients:

1 apple
1 bunch of kale
1 handful of parsley
1-inch piece of ginger root
2 carrots, peeled and ends cut off
1 tomato
1/2 head of broccoli
1/2 cucumber
2 stalks of celery

Instructions:
Remove all stems and seeds from fruits and vegetables.
Slowly add all ingredients to juicer and process juice.
Pour into a glass, and add ice if desired.

Nutritional Info:
Calories: 123
Total Fat: 1.2g
Total Carbohydrates: 16.2g
Dietary Fiber: 6.8g
Sugars: 11.2g
Protein: 3.7g
Sodium: 17mg

Bean Power Cleanse

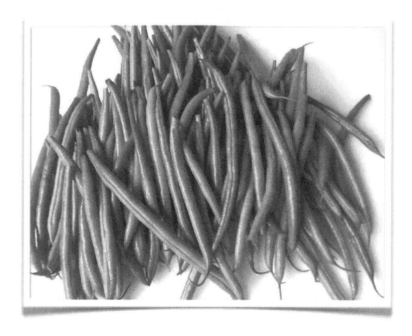

This is a great full-body cleanse recipe that will most likely leave you feeling refreshed and energized. This cleanse has a mixture of great veggies which will undoubtedly cleanse your body of toxins. You can drink this juice at any point during your cleanse.

Start to finish time: 15 minutes

Difficulty Level: Easy

Yield: (1) 8-oz. glass

Ingredients:
2 romaine lettuce leaves
1/2 cucumber
1 large tomato
7-10 string beans, stems removed
1/2 lemon, peeled
1 cup Brussels Sprouts

Instructions:
Bunch lettuce and fit into juicer.
Juice the cucumber next to allow for maximum juice flow.
Add string beans and Brussels sprouts into juicer.
Juice the tomato well, for maximum juice.
Pour into a glass. Add ice, if desired, and serve.

Nutritional info:
Calories: 86
Total Fat: 1.2g
Total Carbohydrates: 14.2g
Dietary Fiber: 5.8g
Sugars: 9.2g
Protein: 3.7g
Sodium: 17mg

The Citrus Green Cleanse

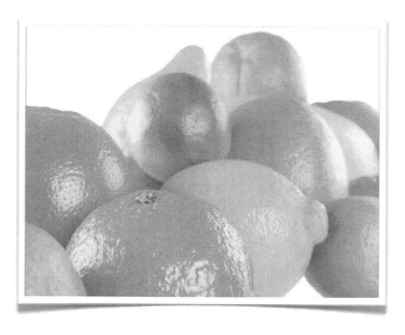

This is a great detox solution with a mix of sweet and natural elements, providing a huge boost of vitamin C and other much-needed nutrients such as chlorophyll, which cleanses the digestive tract.

Start to finish time: 10 minutes

Difficulty Level: Easy

Yield: (1) 8-oz. glass

Ingredients:

6 large green leafy lettuce leaves
Large handful of spinach
1 handful of alfalfa sprouts
2 oranges, peeled and sliced
2 medium sized Tomatoes

Instructions:
Bunch lettuce and fit into juicer.
Process spinach and alfalfa sprouts through the juicer.
Add orange slices to the juicer.
Juice the tomato for maximum juice well.
Pour into a glass. Add ice, if desired, and serve.

Nutritional info:
Calories: 118
Total Fat: 2.3g
Total Carbohydrates: 23.2g
Dietary Fiber: 2.5g
Sugars: 15.2g

The All-Fruit Cleanse

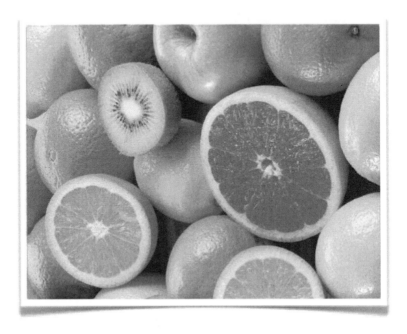

This cleanse will keep you flushed, and is a good break from all the vegetables you'll be doing on the juicing cleanse. It's good to break up the vegetable routine every now and then with an all-fruit recipe. This will keep you satisfied and give you a break from having to add vegetables every time. Note: This should only be done every few days to avoid high-sugar intake and insulin spikes.

Start to finish time: 10 minutes

Difficulty Level: Easy

Yield: (1) 8-oz. glass

Ingredients:
3 apples, washed and cut (remove seeds)
2 cups watermelon, cubed
1 kiwi, peeled
1 lime, peeled

Instructions:
Juice apples first.
Process watermelon, kiwi and lime after.
Pour into a glass. Add ice, if desired, and serve.

Nutritional info:
Calories: 158
Total Fat: 3.2g
Total Carbohydrates: 17.8g
Dietary Fiber: 3g
Sugars: 2.8g
Protein: 1.3g
Sodium: 4mg

Fat-Buster

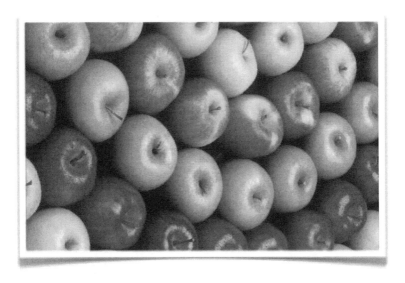

This is a great metabolism booster, with all of your essential ingredients that allow your body to get the optimal amount of necessary vitamins. This particular juice is amazing for a simple metabolism-booster with minimum ingredients.

Start to finish time: 3 - 8 minutes

Difficulty Level: Easy

Yield: (1) 8-oz. glass

Ingredients:
1 1/2 - 2 apples, washed and cut (remove seeds)

1/2 cup seedless grapes
1 teaspoon licorice root powder

Instructions:
Juice apples first.
Juice grapes next.
Stir in licorice powder (do not put in juicer).
Pour into a glass. Add ice, if desired, and serve.

Nutritional info:
Calories: 162
Total Fat: 0.2g
Total Carbohydrates: 14.8g
Dietary Fiber: 4.6g
Sugars: 16.8g
Protein: 0.9g
Sodium: 3.2mg

What To Expect After A Cleanse

After a cleanse, results may vary from individual to individual. However, this typically depends on the toxicity level in your cells and, most of all, how many days you participated in the cleanse. Some individuals will do a cleanse for 3 to 5 days. Others might do a cleanse for one 24-hour period. It all depends on how healthy you are in your normal everyday life. For example, if you eat a lot of fast food or processed foods, you may want to do a 3 to 5 day cleanse.

Here are a few of the good symptoms you may find after doing a cleanse:

Overall improvement in your immune system
Thyroid improvement
An overall increase in energy
Weight loss and fat loss
Lower blood pressure and cholesterol levels
An overall feeling of replenishment

After a juice cleanse, you will notice an almost immediate difference in your skin and overall vitality. It will definitely help you feel more energized!

Food For Thought

Juicing is promoted as an excellent way to cleanse your body of toxins that build up over time. It is estimated that there are between five and ten pounds of old matter in the body. With all this buildup, the body has a hard time keeping a solid routine for digesting food. Start juicing, clean your system, and start feeling great again!

Acceptable Juicing Practices

There are several recommended and popular juice cleanses to consider. Most juice cleanses last from one to five days, with a few longer ones lasting as long as ten days or even more. For convenience, it is a good idea to prepare enough juice for the entire day. I typically juice between 16-32 ounces of fruit and vegetable juice on a daily basis, depending on what I'm trying to accomplish. If I'm doing a juice cleanse, I'll typically drink up to 32 ounces (this equates to four 8-oz. servings per day), but most days I stick to 16 oz. I would suggest using up to 50 percent green "super" vegetables since they are high in chlorophyll and believed to promote healing of the digestive tract.

Certain fruits and vegetables are easier to juice than others. Selecting produce without pits or tough outer skins makes it easier on your juicer. Great choices include apples, carrots, spinach, beets, kale, leafy greens, and celery, to name a few. (Check the chart and recipes for mixing and matching combos.)

Juicing for Weight Loss and Energy - Phase 2 (Maintenance)

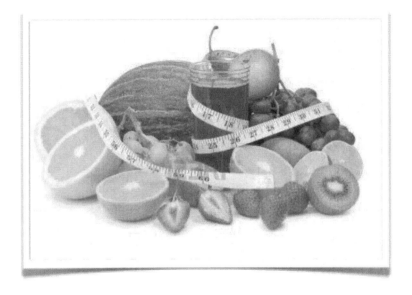

The second phase of your juicing regimen incorporates juicing into your daily routine. This is the time when you go back to eating a balanced diet and (hopefully) replace any bad eating habits you had before with a much more wholesome one! After the cleanse, you will feel lighter, more energetic, and your overall health will feel a ton better! Remember this feeling, and try your best to stay on the proper course. Your body will thank you for it!

Working Out - Physical Activity

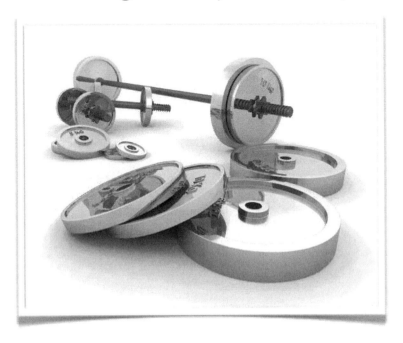

After your detox is over and you begin your juicing routine, it is important to do some basic exercise to keep your metabolism working on all cylinders. This doesn't have to be hard or strenuous! You don't even need to go to the gym! Here are some basic exercises you can do after you wake up and before going to bed at night:

20 Pushups - woman can do pushups with their knees on the floor (go until you feel the burn).
30-40 Air Squats - (go until you feel the burn).

That's it!

Just doing this 3-minute workout before you go to work, or start your day, will jump-start your metabolism. Your juicing routine will then take care of your insides and digestive tract, helping you shed unwanted body fat.

Food For Thought:

Remember, juicing doesn't HAVE to be done every day. What is important is the routine you get yourself in. This way it becomes habit after repetition and scheduled juicing days. I would recommend juicing 3 days a week if every day is too much. Schedule this around your grocery shopping, as it is imperative that you have fresh produce for your juicing days. A typical schedule could look like this:

Monday - Pick up your juicing ingredients for the next three days.

Thursday - Stop by the grocery store for your weekend juicing ingredients.

Typically, try to avoid buying more than 3 days' worth of juicing ingredients at any one given time. This will insure your ingredients are the freshest possible.

Herbs for Weight Loss

When juicing, it is important to know that using certain herbs can also help aid in the weight loss process. Here are two I love using in my daily juicing:

Yerba Mate and Guarana - These are two of my favorite herbs, mainly because they add to your energy levels throughout the day. Yerba Mate, especially, is amazing because it has antioxidant properties as well as a natural source of caffeine. It's good because it gives a burst of energy without the dreaded crash of coffee.

Ginseng - This is an awesome herb that has some serious health benefits. It helps type 2 diabetes, helps with weight loss control, acts as a physical and mental health stimulant, and can also prove to help reproductive systems function better (male sexual functioning and female menstrual cramps).

Phase 2 Recipes (Maintenance)

Phase 2 recipes were designed to help you maintain your juicing routine and incorporate them into your everyday life. Once again, there isn't an exact science to this phase, but these recipes should help you each day. Usually people find a few they really like and stick with them.

Tomato Garden Delight

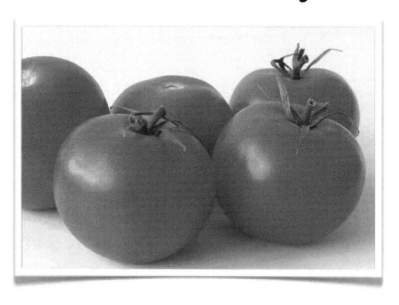

This juice is great because it has the ability to help "fill you up" and cure hunger pangs. Ideally, I would drink something like this in the morning or for an afternoon snack. If you love tomato juice, this may be right up your alley!

Start to finish time: 10 minutes

Difficulty Level: Easy

Yield: (1) 8-oz. glass

Ingredients:

2 medium tomatoes
2 celery sticks
1 large handful of parsley
1 large handful of cilantro
1 medium carrot

Instructions:
Process tomatoes, parsley, cilantro in juicer.
Next add carrots, and finally, celery last.
Pour into a glass. Add ice, if desired, and serve.

Nutritional info:
Calories: 158
Total Fat: 2.2g
Total Carbohydrates: 20.8g
Dietary Fiber: 3g
Sugars: 8.8g
Protein: 1.3g
Sodium: 4.5mg

Watermelon Tango

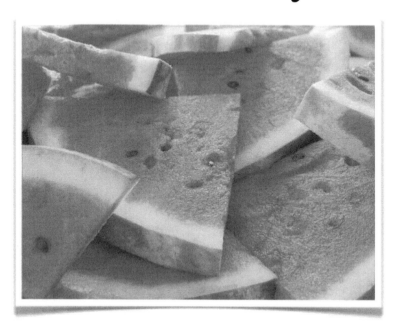

This is a refreshing, delightful beverage that allows for hydration and allows the replenishing of essential electrolytes back into the body. It will also increase your immune system and help flush your digestive tract.

Start to finish time: 10 minutes

Difficulty Level: Easy

Yield: (1) 8-oz. glass

Ingredients:
1 apple
1 cup of watermelon cubes (no seeds)
4 oz. of broccoli
1 handful of watercress

Instructions:
Process apple, watermelon, broccoli, and
watercress into juicer.
Pour into a glass. Add ice, if desired, and serve.

Nutritional info:
Calories: 113
Total Fat: 4.9g
Total Carbohydrates: 17.3g
Dietary Fiber: 4.7g
Sugars: 7.8g
Protein: 2.7g
Sodium: 4.1mg

Veggie Ginger Surprise

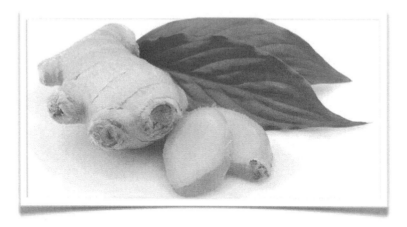

This is a great veggie blend that will clean out your digestive tract. It also focuses on colon and liver health by utilizing several detoxing properties in the greens and beet.

Start to finish time: 10 minutes

Difficulty Level: Easy

Yield: (1) 8-oz. glass

Ingredients:
1 beet
1 green apple
4 large stalks celery
1 large handful of spinach

1 small cucumber
1-inch knob ginger

Instructions:
Process all veggies and fruit through the juicer.
Pour into a glass. Add ice, if desired, and serve.

Nutritional info:
Calories: 120
Total Fat: 3.3g
Total Carbohydrates: 18.3g
Dietary Fiber: 2.3g
Sugars: 9.5g
Protein: 2.5g
Sodium: 3.1mg

The Health Freak

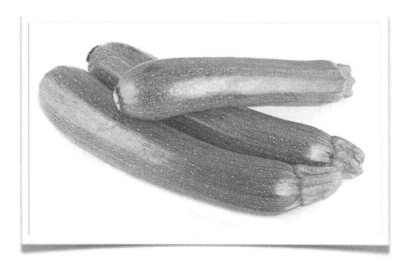

This is a great blend of vegetables and fruits, and contains loads of antioxidants. Antioxidants help rebuild your cells and fight free radicals within your body. Drink this juice and feel a jolt of energy throughout your day!

Start to finish time: 10 minutes

Difficulty Level: Easy

Yield: (1) 8-oz. glass

Ingredients:
2 small zucchini (baby marrow or courgette)

1/4 to 1/2 small purple (red) cabbage, according to taste
2 red apples
4 green or purple kale leaves
4 white or purple cauliflower florets
1 cup blueberries
1 orange, peeled (never juice with skin)
1/2 medium cucumber

Instructions:
Wash and prepare all veggies and fruits.
Discard any skin and seeds accordingly.
Put veggies and fruit through the processor.
Pour into a glass. Add ice, if desired, and serve.

Nutritional info:
Calories: 126
Total Fat: 3.3g
Total Carbohydrates: 18.3g
Dietary Fiber: 2.3g
Sugars: 9.5g
Protein: 2.5g
Sodium: 3.1mg

Green and Mean

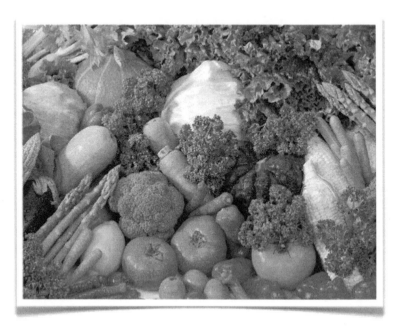

This little treat is high in fiber and low in calories - perfect for incorporating into your everyday juicing. It doesn't fall short of nutrients and vitamins, and it actually fills you up a little bit. This juice is packed with all the nutrients you need for the day, and should give you a good burst of energy as well!

Start to finish time: 10 minutes

Difficulty Level: Easy

Yield: (1) 8-oz. glass

Ingredients:
2 cups spinach
2 cups cucumber
1 head of celery
1/2 inch of ginger root
1 bunch parsley
2 apples
1 lime
1/2 lemon

Instructions:
Wash and prepare all veggies and fruits.
Discard any skin and seeds accordingly.
Put veggies and fruit through the processor.
Pour into a glass. Add ice, if desired, and serve.

Nutritional info:
Calories: 106
Total Fat: 2.3g
Total Carbohydrates: 18.3g
Dietary Fiber: 2.7g
Sugars: 6.5g
Protein: 3.5g
Sodium: 4.1mg

Tomato Filler

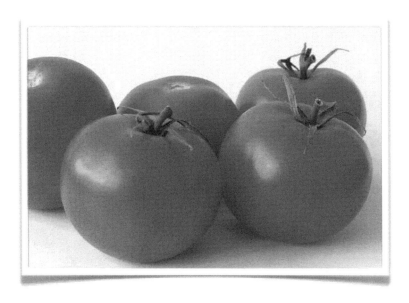

This juicing recipe is designed to act more like a small meal. It is veggie-heavy, so just remember that when you start to make it. If you like tomatoes, you're going to like this recipe. The lemon will help mask some of the "vegetable" taste. I personally find this particular juice very refreshing. :)

Start to finish time: 10 minutes

Difficulty Level: Easy

Yield: (1) 8-oz. glass

Ingredients:
2 medium tomatoes
2 large carrots
1 cup of parsley
2 celery stalks
1/4 lemon
1/2 Cucumber

Instructions:
Cut carrots and cucumbers into smaller pieces and feed into your juicer.
Add Tomatoes, parsley, and celery.
Add lemon to the juicer.
After juicing, pour into a glass. Add ice, if desired, and serve.

Nutritional info:
Calories: 122
Total Fat: 1.7g
Total Carbohydrates: 23.5g
Dietary Fiber: 9.1g
Sugars: 15.1g
Protein: 3.2g
Sodium: 172mg

Kale Surprise

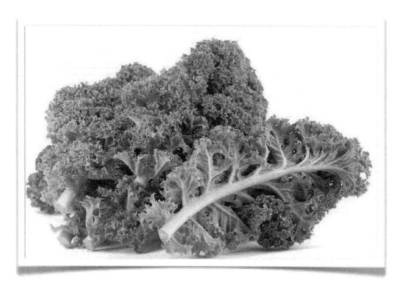

Kale is one of the most nutrient-dense foods you can eat, and it is a must in any juicer's arsenal. The taste is just ok, but when coupled with a fruit like an apple, the taste doesn't become an issue. Kale is amazing - it is high in enzymes, low in fat, and high in fiber. Kale is also high in vitamin K and antioxidants, so drinking this juice will seriously do your body good!

Start to finish time: 10 minutes

Difficulty Level: Easy

Yield: (1) 8-oz. glass

Ingredients:
3 carrots
1 apple
3-4 celery stalks
3 cups of kale

Instructions:
Wash and prepare all veggies and fruits.
Discard any skin and seeds accordingly.
Put veggies and fruit through the processor.
Pour into a glass. Add ice, if desired, and serve.

Nutritional info:
Calories: 111
Total Fat: 1.3g
Total Carbohydrates: 14.3g
Dietary Fiber: 5.7g
Sugars: 3.4g
Protein: 3.5g
Sodium: 3.1mg

Juicing Considerations

Strenuous exercise is not recommended during a
cleanse. Lighter exercise, like walking, is a good
substitute for bolstering circulation and blood-

flow. Depending on how energetic a person feels during a fast, other forms of activity, like tennis or golf, are also good choices.

For some people, juicing will leave you feeling hungry. Should hunger pangs become too bothersome, then partaking in some vegetable broth, fruit or a fresh salad is recommended. Eating a healthy snack like the ones mentioned above will serve to keep the cleanse process in motion without doing any damage.

Conclusion

Juicing has been embraced as an excellent way to promote healing. The many benefits make the effort worthwhile, and I hope you have learned something through reading this book. There are so many benefits to juicing - including improvements in mental function, vital organs, energy levels, digestion, mood, weight, hair and skin. I want to thank you for taking the time to learn something that will improve your life.

With all of the garbage food in the world, we encourage you to bring it back to nature and feed yourself whole foods filled with essential vitamins and nutrients.

Would You Do Me A Quick Favor?

If you liked this book and/or found it helpful, (liked a recipe, learned something new, etc), I would really appreciate it if you left a review on Amazon for me. Trust me... your support on Amazon means the world to me! It really helps me out, and I read every single review.

Just click this link 48 hours after purchasing and click the button that says "create your own review" at the top of the page. Takes 1 minute. Thank you so much! :)

>>Click Here To Leave Review<<

More Amazon Best Sellers That Compliment Juicing:

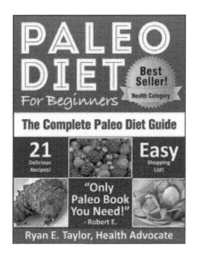

Go Here -- FCRW.org/paleo

Made in the USA
San Bernardino, CA
03 April 2014